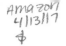

CAREER AS AN

OCCUPATIONAL THERAPIST

THERAPY ASSISTANT

OCCUPATIONAL THERAPY IS ONE OF the hottest careers in healthcare. There are plenty of opportunities, and the need is growing for occupational therapists (and occupational therapy assistants and aides) all over the country. In fact, the number of jobs is predicted to swell by 30 percent over the next 10 years.

What is occupational therapy? It is a health and rehabilitation profession providing services for people of all ages who may need help to lead productive, independent, and fulfilling lives. Patients may need specialized assistance as a result of physical, developmental, social, or emotional problems. The term "occupational" does not only relate to jobs, but may include any task or activity, whether it is work-related, recreational, or part of daily life, such as getting dressed, cooking, and driving. Occupational therapy is a patient-centered practice that relies on holistic principles to assess and treat people as unique individuals. Every treatment plan is designed for a particular patient to help the person achieve specific goals.

Most occupational therapists work in hospitals, skilled nursing facilities, doctors' offices, and schools. A growing number work for home health agencies, providing services to patients in their homes.

Occupational therapists can be generalists, working with people of all ages and with every kind of disability. Being a generalist has its advantages, like keeping every day interesting and providing a wide variety of experiences. Also consider that this is a very flexible career with many different kinds of practice to choose from for those with particular interests. For example, some OTs may enjoy working with school children with Down syndrome or helping amputees regain skills needed to get back to work. Others may prefer to work with premature babies in a pediatric hospital, help veterans with PTSD, or assist older people in nursing homes deal with Alzheimer's disease. There are currently nine specialty areas that offer opportunities for certification. There are also new specialties that do not yet offer certification, but may in the near future. They include autism sensory integration, corrective medicine, and occupational science.

A master's degree is required to become a licensed occupational therapist. If an individual is not ready to invest the money and time (six years on average following high school graduation), there are alternatives. It only takes a two-year associate degree to be eligible for certification as an occupational therapy assistant (COTA). COTAs do much the same work as occupational therapists, and they are paid quite well considering the modest educational requirements. A COTA's average annual salary is about $60,000, which is about 70 percent of what a licensed occupational therapist can expect.

Someone wishing to enter the field can also qualify for a job as an occupational therapy aide with no more than a high school diploma. People who start out as assistants or aides usually go back to school at some point to do the additional work required to become an occupational therapist.

Occupational therapy can offer a lifetime career that is challenging and diversified. If you are looking for a career in the healthcare field that offers satisfying and rewarding work, read on.

WHAT YOU CAN DO NOW

THE EDUCATION REQUIRED IS A BIG commitment if you are not absolutely sure this is the right career for you. If you are considering this career, take some time to explore the field as soon as possible. The best way to start is to talk to professionals who are actually working in occupational therapy. Ask your guidance counselor to invite professionals to speak at your school on career days or help arrange job-shadowing opportunities. Spending a day or two with an occupational therapist is a great way to learn what you can expect to be doing on a daily basis. Be prepared to ask intelligent questions and get advice on how best to prepare.

Another good way to test the waters is by working as an occupational therapy aide. You only need a high school diploma or GED to land a job as an aide. No special training is required other than what your employer will provide on the job. Look for volunteer work as an aide. Many college OT programs expect applicants to have volunteered. It is also an excellent way to get a real feel for what this career is like. Aides work closely with the occupational therapists and often do very similar work. Ideally, you will find an opportunity in a clinical environment, such as a hospital or occupational therapy clinic.

Be prepared to pursue college and graduate school education. If you determine that this is the right career for you, you will want to be ready to start your higher education right away. Research admission requirements and start preparing your application materials. Any college OT program will include numerous science courses. In high school, the best subjects to focus on are biology, anatomy, and psychology. Take advanced courses if they are available. Any classes involving health and wellness will also be beneficial. Be sure to keep your grades up. Admission officers will expect to see a GPA of at least 3.0.

HISTORY OF THE PROFESSION

MANY PEOPLE BELIEVE THAT OCCUPATIONAL therapy is a new profession. In fact, it began 100 years ago. The philosophies and methodologies that comprise the building blocks of the profession started to emerge in the 1700s, but occupational therapy began as a profession in 1917 (though it was not officially named that until 1920).

It was in 1917 that five people came together to found what is now known as the American Occupational Therapy Association (AOTA). The purpose of the organization then and now is to represent the interests and concerns of occupational therapy practitioners and students, and improve the quality of occupational therapy services. Among the founding members, there were three individuals who played pivotal roles: William Rush Dunton, Jr., Eleanor Clarke Slagle, and Susan Tracy.

William Rush Dunton, Jr. is known as the "father of occupational therapy." He was a psychiatrist and educator who published the first account of the occupational therapy profession. During his work with the mentally ill, he became fascinated with the healing potential of occupational activities for patients, and routinely recommended treatment plans that included emphasis on busy, productive activities in the daily lives of his patients. In 1918, Dunton published a textbook for nurses entitled *Occupational Therapy: A Manual for Nurses.* The manual spelled out how OT should be utilized in clinical settings. That same year his article *The Principles of Occupational Therapy,* published in Public Health magazine, laid the foundation for the textbook to be published in 1919 entitled *Reconstruction Therapy.* In that textbook, he wrote that all patients "should have occupations which they enjoy, that sick minds, sick bodies, and sick souls may be healed through occupation." In a later textbook, *Prescribing Occupational Therapy*, published in 1928, he declared that:

"Occupation is as necessary as food and drink."

Eleanor Clark Slagle, a social worker and early pioneer of occupational therapy, is known as the "mother of occupational therapy." In 1912, Slagle became director of a department of occupational therapy at the Johns Hopkins Hospital – a department she helped create. It was the first professional school for occupational therapy in the US. Up until the founding of AOTA in 1917, occupational therapy had not been taken seriously as a medical career. Having witnessed the healing effects of OT, Slagle was determined to help the profession expand and gain the respect it deserved. She focused her efforts as a charter member of AOTA on promoting the field of occupational therapy as a vital profession. Her efforts did not go unnoticed. During the third annual meeting of AOTA, she was elected president.

AOTA founder, Susan Tracy, is considered the first occupational therapist. As a nurse, she observed the benefits of active occupations in relieving nervous tension and making bed rest more tolerable for patients. Upon noticing that this was particularly true for those who suffered from mental illness, she began to specialize in this field. Tracy is also well known for creating programs designed to educate student nurses on the therapeutic use of activities as part of treatment. Tracy coined the term "Occupational Nurse" for those she successfully trained in this specialty.

As the AOTA was being established, World War I was devastating Europe. The Red Cross realized that occupational therapists would be needed to help World War I veterans adjusting to civilian life upon returning to the United States. There were countless thousands of veterans who needed help, requiring the use of every available therapist possible. AOTA members were called upon to develop programs for treating injured soldiers. In 1941, the United States again found itself involved in a World War. During the war, OT services continued to grow, especially among military hospitals. By the end of the war, there were 21

OT programs and 3224 occupational therapists. There were also more than five million people who needed care!

From the 1940s through the 1960s, the "Rehabilitation Movement" helped the growth of the profession and increased public awareness of the benefits of occupational therapy. Thousands of injured soldiers returning home from war created a surge in the demand for OT services. OTs who had previously treated only the institutionalized mentally ill, began treating physical disabilities due to the injuries sustained in battle. As the focus shifted away from mental illness, more and more types of physical disabilities were treated, including spinal cord injuries, amputations, traumatic brain injuries, and cerebral palsy.

In 1956 The Certified Occupational Therapy Assistant (COTA) job role was created to alleviate the demand for OTs. The supply of qualified professional OTs was not keeping up with the demand, mostly due to the education that was required. The COTA required only minimal formal training. Any necessary specific training was provided on the job while working as an assistant or aide to a licensed OT.

The field of occupational therapy continued to grow. During the 1960s, medicine in general became more specialized. Occupational therapists began to specialize, too, particularly in the areas of pediatrics and developmental disabilities.

The Rehabilitation Act of 1973 was a landmark legislation that prohibited discrimination against people with disabilities. It was followed by the passing of the Individual With Disabilities Education Act in 1975. When this Act was introduced, the public was becoming more educated about disabilities and more accepting of people with disabilities. Even before these laws, schools were becoming more accommodating for students with disabilities, hiring more occupational therapists to help students of all ages in educational settings.

As the end of the 20th century neared, occupational therapy

began to focus more on a person's quality of life. Occupation therapy started to involve more patient education, prevention, screenings, and health maintenance. Today, occupational therapy is still evolving as a dynamic profession. Occupational therapists can be found working in widely diverse settings, providing vital services to people of all ages and disabilities.

WHERE YOU WILL WORK

OCCUPATIONAL THERAPISTS CAN BE found in many different employment environments, including hospitals, rehabilitation centers, schools, small medical offices, and clients' homes. Some also work in policy and administration, as well as research and academia. It is common for OTs to work in multiple facilities and to travel from one job to another.

There are about 115,000 occupational therapists working in the US. The percentage of occupational therapists working for the largest employers is as follows:

- Hospitals (state, local, and private)   28 %

- Private practices of physical, occupational, and speech therapists   22 %

- Elementary and secondary schools, both public and private   12 %

- Skilled nursing facilities   9 %

- Home healthcare services   9%

Most people are introduced to occupational therapy in a hospital. While acute care in a hospital setting may be the starting point for therapy, hospital care is very short term in nature. Patients who are admitted to a hospital may work briefly with an occupational therapist to get help recovering from a physical trauma. The goal in this case is for the patient to recover as quickly as possible in preparation for discharge. Any care provided beyond this would be considered long-term rehabilitation and would require extended services beyond the hospital environment.

Long-term care is usually provided in an in-patient rehabilitation facility. In this case, the patient would undergo intensive therapy, with treatment often lasting for several hours per day. Patients in this setting are expected to recover at some point. The OT's goal is to help them become self-sufficient so they can eventually go home and live a normal life.

Another form of extended care is provided in nursing homes for the elderly or developmentally disabled. In this setting, patients are not necessarily expected to recover from any sort of illness or injury. Instead, they are permanent residents in these facilities and their work with occupational therapists is ongoing. In this setting, the OT's job is to manage the patient's condition, not cure it.

A growing number of OTs work for home health agencies. There are times when home healthcare is needed for patients who have limited mobility and/or cannot fully function independently. In this case, the occupational therapist would travel to the patient's home to provide care.

There is also a wide variety of alternative clinical settings where occupational therapists can be found. Because occupational therapists work with people of all ages and developmental abilities, they can choose their work setting based on their area of expertise or interest. Some of the alternative settings where occupational therapists work include:

- Corporate employee health centers

- Government health agencies

- Organizations for the handicapped

- Adult day care centers

- Community health centers

In settings such as these, the duties of the occupational therapist would be entirely based on the needs of the employer.

Some OTs prefer the flexibility of being self-directed. In fact, almost 10 percent of all occupational therapists are self-employed. They may work from their own home and use part of their own residence as office space. Some choose to utilize some sort of treatment facility as a place to meet with their clients. A growing number of independent OTs receive work assignments through locum tenens (temporary) staffing agencies.

Work Schedules

Most occupational therapists work full time. About 30 percent work part time. Occupational therapists in hospitals and other healthcare and community settings typically work a 40-hour week. They may work nights or weekends, as needed, to accommodate the schedules of individual patients. Occupational therapists who work in schools may need to stay after school for meetings or other activities.

THE WORK YOU WILL DO

OCCUPATIONAL THERAPISTS HELP people of all ages develop, recover, and improve the skills needed for daily living. Patients may need help temporarily during recovery from injury, surgery, or illness. Others may be permanently disabled, mentally ill, or dealing with chronic conditions such as diabetes, cerebral palsy, or autism. Regardless of the issue, the OT's job is to help people do the everyday "occupations" of life such as getting dressed, cooking, bathing, operating a computer, and driving.

Every new patient is thoroughly evaluated before proceeding with treatment. Assessment includes both the patient and the patient's work and home environment. Occupational therapists take a holistic approach, focusing on adapting the environment to fit the person rather than the other way around. It is particularly important that the OT understand the patient's goals in order to create an effective plan. Every patient is unique and every treatment plan is customized specifically to the needs of each individual. To accomplish this, occupational therapists follow a basic routine:

- Review patient's medical history and evaluate their current condition

- Evaluate patient's home and/or workplace and identify areas of potential improvements, such as labeling kitchen cabinets for an older person with poor memory

- Observe the individual doing tasks and determine specific needs

- Develop a treatment plan that defines the types of activities and specific goals to be accomplished

- Recommend special equipment, such as wheelchairs and

eating aids

- Demonstrate exercises and how to use assistive devices

- Educate patient's family, teachers, and/or employer about how to accommodate and care for the patient

- Keep meticulous records of patient's activities and progress

- OTs also oversee the work of occupational therapy assistants and aides.

Occupational therapists are an integral part of a healthcare team, which may include doctors, registered nurses, and other kinds of therapists.

Specialties

As in most healthcare fields, occupational therapy provides opportunities to specialize. There are currently nine areas in which an occupational therapist can become certified as a specialist.

Gerontology

This is a huge area for occupational therapists. Those who work with the elderly help their patients lead more independent and active lives, whether they are recovering from strokes or dealing with Alzheimer's disease. According to the AOTA, "productive aging" is a key practice area within the specialty. The need for OTs in this area results from increased longevity, the changing world of work, and especially baby boomers' focus on quality of life. OTs help seniors who are experiencing age-related physical limitations re-engage in activities they love, such as sports and travel.

Pediatrics

Working exclusively with children is another thriving area for occupational therapy. Pediatric OTs help kids fully engage in the "occupations" of childhood – learning, playing, and growing. That generally means helping kids experience the pleasure of successful play, self-care, and socializing. Some practitioners concentrate on subspecialties such as early intervention therapy for infants and toddlers who are at risk of having developmental delays, or working with premature babies or children with cerebral palsy, autism, or Down syndrome.

Mental Health

Practice in this area is focused on helping patients who suffer from developmental disabilities, mental illness, or emotional problems. Patients with developmental issues may need to learn how to budget, use public transportation, or do household chores. The specialty also deals with drug abuse, alcoholism, depression, and other disorders. OTs also work with people who have been through a traumatic event.

Physical Rehabilitation

Practitioners in this area typically choose to help accident victims restore lost function and regain needed skills for their daily routine at home and at work. There is also a wide variety of issues a physical rehabilitation specialist can address. These include everything from burns to amputations, spinal cord injuries to strokes.

Driving and Community Mobility

OT practitioners in this specialty understand how important it is for people to be able to get around. Specifically, they know how progressive conditions and life changes can affect driving. Changes in physical, mental, and sensory abilities can diminish a person's continued ability to drive safely. This is particularly true for aging adults, which is why most OTs in this specialty spend their time evaluating and training older drivers. They can help people maintain their independence – something that is very important to most people as they get older. This usually means helping them make a smooth transition from driving, to using other forms of transportation without losing their sense of self-worth.

Environmental Modification

Work in this area can take place in the home, school, or workplace. The OT starts with a comprehensive evaluation of the environment, and then either creates a functional environment or recommends changes using adaptive equipment. The OT also provides training and guidance for the patient, family members, caregivers, and employers. Some practitioners subspecialize in office ergonomics. They may make changes to the workplace environment or simply train workers to use the correct ergonomics.

Feeding, Eating, and Swallowing

OT practitioners collaborate with doctors and other types of therapists to help patients with a variety of diagnoses to eat and swallow safely. Treatment may be temporary or continue across a patient's entire life. These specialists are trained to identify problems with the oral, pharyngeal, and esophageal phases of swallowing and provide treatment that will ensure they perform correctly. In addition to diagnosis, the OT's job tasks include setting up special equipment, teaching patients how to do exercises and use equipment, and tracking eating habits to ensure that nutritional guidelines are being met.

Low Vision

People can experience low vision for a number of reasons, including injury, disease, or simply the consequence of aging. Whatever the case, OT specialists can help people with low vision maintain their independence, participate in daily activities, function at the highest level possible, and avoid accidents. Therapy is usually only needed when vision problems cannot be corrected with eyeglasses, contact lenses, or surgery. Treatment ranges from the basics (improved lighting or recommending magnifiers) to teaching new skills, such as eccentric viewing or visual tracking.

School Systems

A growing number of occupational therapists specialize in working with children in educational settings. Therapy may be provided anywhere in the school environment, including the classroom, library, cafeteria, playground, or other designated areas. The work involves evaluating disabled children's abilities, modifying classroom equipment to accommodate them, and helping them to participate in school activities. Specific tasks may include working on fine motor skills such as handwriting, helping a student with time management, or adapting learning materials to facilitate success in school. OTs work with students who have learning disabilities, behavioral problems, or autism.

Certified Occupational Therapist Assistant (COTA)

Occupational therapy assistants, or COTAs, work under the direct supervision of an occupational therapist. They do much of the same work that occupational therapists do and the work environment is identical, whether it takes place in a hospital or in a patient's home. Routine tasks typically include moving patients, setting up equipment or materials, explaining exercises, and writing reports on patient treatment. What an occupational therapy assistant is not permitted to do is diagnose illnesses and formulate a treatment plan without supervision by an occupational therapist.

Occupational Therapy Aide

Occupational therapy aides are entry-level members of the occupational therapy team. They work full time or part time under the direct supervision of an occupational therapist or occupational therapy assistant. They are usually employed in hospitals or physician offices, but it is also common for them to accompany their supervising OT or COTA to the homes of patients.

Typical job duties of an aide may include:

- Helping patients fill out paperwork

- Setting up and putting away therapy equipment

- Cleaning equipment before and after treatment sessions

- Answering phones and scheduling appointments

- Explaining terminology to patients and their families

Usually, only a COTA will help assist with a patient's treatment. But occasionally, an aide may be asked to help move a patient or help keep a patient steady during an exercise.

OCCUPATIONAL THERAPY PROS TELL THEIR OWN STORIES

I Help People Do What They Love Most

"I didn't start out wanting to be an occupational therapist. I wanted to help people and was always interested in the mind-body connection. I thought being a psychologist was the obvious choice, but I discovered in a discussion with my faculty advisor that occupational therapy embraces that holistic approach more than any other field. In OT, it is used systematically to help people accomplish their goals. The mind-body connection simply means you can learn to use your thoughts to positively influence your body's physical responses. When I realized OT was a field in which I could see results that are more tangible from my work, I was sold.

There is a common misconception about the field of occupational therapy. People often assume it's about helping people find jobs or retraining because they can no longer work in their profession for some reason. But the word ".occupation" in this field refers to any activity or task that people do every day, whether it's in the workplace, at home, or elsewhere. If you think about it, human life comprises hundreds of daily activities that occupy our waking hours.

Another misconception is that our work is focused on healing some physical ailment that is restricting the patient's ability to perform. The fact is, we don't ask 'what's the matter with you.' Instead, we ask 'what matters to you?' While a physical therapist might help someone to walk after an injury, an occupational therapist might help that person to dance. It doesn't matter if we are helping to develop new abilities or restore some that have been lost or diminished. As an OT therapist, I work with whatever issues the patient is dealing with. It could be mental, physical, emotional, developmental, or any combination.

It's an exciting time to be an occupational therapist. The field is continually changing and advancing. One of the most interesting changes in the field has been the introduction of occupational science. That is the scientific study of the phenomena of human activity. It is an academic discipline focused on the impact of occupation on the health of individuals and communities. The work of occupational scientists validates and supports what we do as clinical occupational therapists.

It is a great time to become an occupational therapist. There is immediate demand for our services, especially since millions of baby boomers are striving to maintain their independence and active lifestyles. In fact, occupational therapy is one of the fastest growing careers, and it is almost recession-proof. Job security is great, yet the field has so much more to offer. Every day I make a positive impact on other people's lives. I can't imagine a more satisfying career. Anyone who is interested in helping people should take a look. Being an occupational therapist has changed my life. It could change yours, too."

I Am an Occupational Therapy Assistant

"I became interested in occupational therapy after observing how much it helped my sister after having breast cancer. I researched the requirements to enter the field and quickly realized that I was not in a position to commit to six years of college. I expressed my disappointment to my sister's OT, and she urged me to consider starting out as an assistant. The education would only take two years, and I could take classes at night, leaving me free to continue working my day job. That's what I did, and it was the best decision I've ever made.

I work in a VA hospital doing inpatient rehabilitation. Unlike most COTAs, I don't see a lot of different patients throughout the day. Instead, I have maybe five or six patients that I work with over a long period of time. I might spend an hour or two with each patient every day for six months to a year, helping these soldiers practice new skills in their hospital room. Treatment varies from patient to patient, but my goal is always the same – return the person to the functional level of life before being injured. That doesn't mean the patient will be the same. There may be a missing limb or a brain injury. The patient has to understand that many things will not be done in quite the same way as before the injury. I will teach alternative ways to accomplish daily tasks such as bathing, brushing teeth, getting dressed, and cooking. A successful treatment plan eventually helps the patient become independent and fully engaged in life again.

What I like best about my work is seeing the patient progress and return to normal life. It is extremely rewarding. When I see new patients, they are at the lowest points in their life. They are often depressed, sometimes even suicidal. A big part of my job is to give them hope and encourage them through months of painstaking hard work. It can be heartbreaking at times, but I know I have the skills to help them, and that one day I will be able to give their life back. I don't think I've ever finished a last session that didn't end with hugs and tears of gratitude. I can't think of another career where I could make such a difference in a person's life."

PERSONAL QUALIFICATIONS

WHILE STUDYING TO BECOME AN occupational therapist, having a head for science and math will certainly help you to understand how the human body works. Beyond school, there is a much larger array of vital personal skills needed to succeed in this career.

Compassion

Occupational therapists are typically attracted to the profession because they want to help people. The best OTs are naturally nurturing and have a genuine interest in helping others live more active and fulfilling lives. Their dedication to that end is unwavering as they work with people through obstacles to find solutions.

Communications Skills

In this profession, communication starts with listening. Occupational therapists must be able to listen attentively to what patients tell them so they fully understand what the goals are. You must always take patients seriously – what is important to one person may be totally different than anyone else. Excellent speaking skills are needed to clearly explain the treatment plan to patients and their families. Good written communication skills are also necessary. Keeping track of patient progress is a big part of the job. It does not involve a lot of time, but it is important to record accurate notes after every session and write reports on patients' progress.

Interpersonal Skills

Are you a people person? Being around people and working with people – all sorts of people – that is what you do as an OT. Because occupational therapy is centered on people, empathy and strong social skills are important. Occupational therapy is as much mental as it is physical. A positive attitude and optimism are needed to encourage patients to keep going. Therapy is not easy. Patients often struggle with difficult tasks and exercises. A therapist's positive attitude can go a long way toward motivating and encouraging patients to work through it and realize their goals.

Patience

Dealing with any kind of disability is naturally frustrating for many people. Some will take their frustrations out on you. You will need to have more patience than they do, to be able to remain calm and continually offer reassurance. Therapy regimens can be painful and tedious. It is not unusual for patients to want to give up. This can take its toll on you emotionally, so learning how to handle stress is important.

Flexibility

Not every type of therapy will work for each patient. Figuring out the best therapy prescription for patients is not always easy to accomplish. Occupational therapists must be creative when determining the treatment plans and adaptive devices that best suit each patient's needs. It is important to remain flexible. If progress is not being made, you will need to adapt and apply your own ingenuity to suit a patient's particular needs and circumstances. The most successful occupational therapists have a unique combination of critical thinking ability, manual skills, and emotional intelligence.

ATTRACTIVE FEATURES

SURVEYS HAVE REVEALED THAT OCCUPATIONAL therapists are very happy with their career choice. It is not surprising considering the plethora of benefits. Some of the favorites cited include virtually endless job opportunities, numerous different places to practice, opportunity for creativity, good pay, and rewarding work. These and other advantages make it one of the best careers there is.

Tangible Results

Occupational therapists not only get to see progress, real visible progress, they are part of making that progress happen. No matter how big or small the results may be, this is perhaps the most exciting part of working as an OT. In fact, it is sometimes the tiniest baby steps forward that evoke the biggest thrills. Imagine seeing a patient putting on his shoes all by himself for the first time since having a stroke. Or being in the classroom to witness an autistic student sit fully engaged for all of circle time instead of wandering around the room, or running and hiding under a desk. These are the kinds of tangible results OTs live for.

Creativity

Occupational therapy is an interesting blend of art and science. OTs get to utilize both sides of their brain while seeking creative ways to develop and implement approaches to help patients reach their individual goals. While some practice settings provide more opportunities for creativity than others do, all rely on the therapist's ability to apply knowledge of science and human development to make the most effective body/mind connections.

Flexibility

While most occupational therapists (about 70 percent) work full time, this is one of the few healthcare fields that provide ample opportunities to obtain a good balance between one's professional and personal life. In fact, working part time is becoming increasingly popular and easily attainable. Some part-time therapists work two or three days a week on a regular schedule. Others choose PRN work. PRN is a Latin phrase, *pro re nata*, which means "when necessary." PRN work is typically assigned through tenens locum (temporary) agencies. Therapists signed up with these agencies can pick and choose when and how much they want to work. Not all are part-time workers. Some are full-time therapists who like to earn some extra pay for working a Saturday or holiday here and there. The extra cash is significant, too. The PRN hourly rate is often twice the regular hourly rate for a salaried employee. Do you want to travel? Tenens locums agencies can place you in hospitals or clinics around the US for a few weeks or a few months. It is a great way to see the world while continuing to collect paychecks.

There is also tremendous flexibility in practice settings. OTs can choose to specialize and work only with kids or mental health patients, for example. Or they can get a stimulating mix of everything in one job by working in an acute care hospital setting. There is no reason to ever burn out because there are so many different types of settings to choose from. Tired of working in the school system? Your skills can easily transfer to a number of different employers – a doctor's office, corporation, or branch of government. You can also choose to visit patients in their homes rather than reporting to the same workplace every day.

Excellent Job Outlook

Occupational therapists enjoy exceptional job security. Licensed professionals are needed everywhere and the demand is growing fast. Whether you want to stay in your hometown or move someplace new, you can count on finding a position. Wherever you go, there will always be people who need your help.

UNATTRACTIVE ASPECTS

WHILE OCCUPATIONAL THERAPY MAY be a dream job for many, working in the healthcare field is not for everyone. Not everyone has a head for science and math. Nor is everyone an outgoing person who loves interacting with many different people. Some enter the field with the best of intentions only to discover they are not comfortable dealing with certain bodily functions.

The education required to become a licensed occupational therapist is significant. It typically takes six years to complete. That represents time and expense, and make no mistake, the programs are tough. Prospective OTs should be sure they are prepared to handle all of the clinical and laboratory studies that are coming their way.

An OT's work can certainly be rewarding, but it can also be emotionally draining. It can be stressful dealing with the pain and suffering of patients every day. Not everyone is emotionally up to the challenge. Treatment often goes on over a long period of time – months, years, or even a patient's lifetime. Throughout that time, the OT's positive attitude must never waver. A big part of the job is to continually encourage and reassure patients, no matter how frustrating the situation gets. Learning to deal with the stress will help your own health and well-being.

In some settings, OTs have to rein in their creativity. Insurance companies (Medicare in particular) are very particular about what they will pay for and will insist you strictly follow their guidelines. OTs like being patient-centered, but that can be hard when insurers will not reimburse for treatments you feel would be the most effective.

Some employers have productivity requirements. That often means having to limit the time spent with each patient.

COTAs

Occupational therapy assistants have the advantage of entering their careers much faster than OTs. It only takes two years to prepare for that first job. The pay can be quite generous, considering such a short training period. There are drawbacks though. As an assistant, you do not have much say about what and how treatment will be administered. Your supervising occupational therapist will tell you what to do and you will need to strictly follow all the rules.

While COTAs do much of the same work as OTs, there are limitations. For example, COTAs may not be able to order new tests, complete comprehensive patient assessments, or evaluate home or work environments.

Occupational therapists enjoy a great deal of flexibility in scheduling. COTAs are not always so fortunate. Especially for new COTAs, schedules may have to be part time or on a rotation. It can be difficult to adjust to such an indefinite schedule. For most assistants, the job revolves around the patient. A COTA's schedule may be a mix of weekends, evenings, and early mornings. How crazy a schedule gets depends largely on the work setting. Those who work in nursing homes, schools, and hospitals may have more of a consistent schedule.

EDUCATION AND TRAINING

OCCUPATIONAL THERAPISTS NEED AT least a master's degree in occupational therapy. A growing number of licensed OTs also have a doctoral degree. Occupational therapy programs are accredited by the Accreditation Council for Occupational Therapy Education, which is an arm of the American Occupational Therapy Association. There are currently 149 accredited programs, including 145 master's degree programs and 4 doctoral degree programs.

Admission to master's degree programs in occupational therapy generally requires a bachelor's degree. There is no undergraduate degree in occupational therapy. The American Occupational Therapy Association suggests a variety of appropriate majors that have proven to provide good preparation for graduate studies. The most common include psychology, anthropology, biology, sociology, and kinesiology. Regardless of which major you choose, you will need to include some specific courses, such as biology and physiology. Many OT programs also require some experience working in an occupational therapy setting. Both paid and volunteer work are acceptable.

It generally takes two years of full-time study at the graduate level to earn a master's degree in occupational therapy. There are part-time programs available that offer classes on weekends and nights. This is convenient for people who work regular jobs during the day, but it does extend the time needed for completion to about three years. Those who want to get their careers going as quickly as possible should look for schools that offer an accelerated dual-degree program. In this kind of program, a student can earn both a bachelor's degree and a master's degree in just five years total, instead of the usual six.

Coursework for graduate students is intense and focuses entirely on the practice of occupational therapy. Classes cover every aspect of the field, including a wide array of topics such as functional anatomy, medical and social conditions, assistive technology, patient care concepts, and research methods.

Outside the classroom, students gain clinical work experience through fieldwork in a variety of practice settings. This is not only an essential component of the curriculum, it is required for licensure. Fieldwork is conducted in the same places that most licensed OTs work: rehabilitation centers, nursing homes, acute hospital settings, school systems, and private practices. The average amount of time spent completing fieldwork is 24 weeks.

Licenses and Certifications

All states require occupational therapists to be licensed. To become licensed, candidates must first earn a degree from an accredited educational program, complete all fieldwork requirements, and pass the national examination administered by the National Board for Certification in Occupational Therapy (NBCOT). Successful passage of the exam qualifies therapists to use the title Occupational Therapist Registered (OTR). To maintain certification, licensed OTs must take continuing education classes.

Beyond the basic licensing, there are opportunities to become certified in a number of specialty areas, such as mental health, school systems, or physical rehabilitation. The American Occupational Therapy Association currently offers nine certifications for occupational therapists who want to demonstrate their advanced level of knowledge in a particular area of practice.

Occupational Therapy Assistant Education and Licensure

The American Occupational Therapy Association also regulates educational curriculum and licensure for occupational therapy assistants (COTAs). Licensing is available in all 50 states, the District of Columbia, and Puerto Rico.

To become an occupational therapy assistant, one must first attend an AOTA-accredited college or university. The primary requirement for admission to an associate degree program is a high school diploma or GED equivalent. However, entry for OTA programs is often competitive because class sizes are very small – typically only a dozen or so students. Most OTA programs involve two years of rigorous coursework. Once completed, students are eligible to sit for the National Board for Certification in Occupational Therapy (NBCOT) exam. Passing this exam is required in order to become a Certified Occupational Therapy Assistant (COTA).

Occupational Therapy Aide Options

While there are training programs available for prospective occupational therapy aides, none are accredited by the American Occupational Therapy Association. Attending one of these programs is an unnecessary step to enter the field at this level. You only need a high school diploma or GED equivalent to qualify for most positions. No special training is needed other than that provided on the job. OT aides typically use their training and experience as a springboard to further their careers. Many eventually go back to school and become occupational therapy assistants or occupational therapists.

EARNINGS

THE AVERAGE EARNINGS FOR OCCUPATIONAL therapists have been rising steadily in recent years. It is a matter of supply and demand – the demand for qualified occupational therapists is increasing faster than the supply, putting OTs in a good position to push for higher wages.

The average annual income is now about $77,000, which works out to an hourly wage of $37.00. Only 10 percent earn less than $50,000. The top 10 percent earn more than $108,000.

Salaries do vary by locale and type of employer. The highest pay for OTs is offered in the following five states:

Nevada	$95,000
District of Columbia	$85,000
Texas	$85,000
California	$85,000
New Jersey	$84,000

Most occupational therapists work in one of five settings. Here are the median annual salaries:

Skilled nursing care facilities	$84,000
Home healthcare services	$82,000
Physical, occupational, and speech therapy practices	$77,000
Hospitals (state, local, and private)	$75,000
Elementary and secondary schools (public and private)	$67,000

As you can see, the right combination of location, employer, and experience is the key to higher earnings.

Occupational Therapy Assistant

Occupational therapy assistants earn approximately 70 percent of what occupational therapists earn. That is impressive when you consider COTAs only need a two-year associate degree versus the five or six year master's degree required for most occupational therapists. The average annual salary for COTAs is about $57,000. Nine out of 10 earn more than $37,000, and the top 10 percent earn more than $77,000.

Most COTAs work in private physicians' offices and rehabilitation centers. Those employed in the home healthcare industry (visiting patients in their homes) and nursing care facilities tend to earn more than average. Pay is also generally higher in metropolitan areas.

Occupational Therapy Aide

Income for occupational therapy aides also varies according to location and employer, but it depends on the number of hours worked per week. Unlike OTs and COTAs, occupational therapy aides are often paid hourly wages instead of yearly salaries. Occupational therapy aides are also more likely to work part time.

The average income for occupational therapists aides works out to about $27,000 annually.

OPPORTUNITIES

THE FUTURE LOOKS VERY BRIGHT FOR licensed occupational therapists. Employment in this field is expected to grow nearly 30 percent over the next 10 years. That is much faster than the average for all other occupations.

Occupational therapy will continue to be an important part of treatment for people with all kinds of illnesses and disabilities, both mental and physical. The number one reason so many more occupational therapists are needed now and in the future is the rapidly growing aging population. There are 76 million baby boomers, all of whom are over the age of 50. This is a generation of people who want to remain independent, vital, and active later in life. Occupational therapists can help them do that. OTs routinely treat many conditions and ailments commonly associated with aging, such as arthritis and stroke. Job opportunities should be good for OTs in all settings, but especially in acute hospital, rehabilitation, and orthopedic services, because that is where seniors typically receive treatment.

Occupational therapists will also be needed to treat patients with chronic conditions, such as diabetes, cerebral palsy, and Alzheimer's. A growing number of people are seeking noninvasive outpatient treatment for long-term disabilities and illnesses, either in their homes or in residential care environments. Home healthcare agencies and skilled nursing facilities are among the largest employers of OTs.

Medical advances have also played a role in the increasing demand for occupational therapy services. OTs are now able to help with critical problems such as birth defects or limb amputations. As part of a healthcare team, an occupational therapist can first help the patient survive, then continue treatment to enable patients to perform a variety of daily tasks.

A relatively new and growing area for occupational therapy involves people with autism spectrum disorder. More and more states are requiring insurance companies to cover treatment for autism. Occupational therapy in this area is usually provided through schools, where OTs help kids with autism improve their social skills and accomplish other tasks as well.

The best job prospects are available for occupational therapists with specialized knowledge in a treatment area. There are currently nine specialties in which OTs can become certified. Many OTs choose to narrow their focus within a certified specialty. For example, an OT might be certified for Physical Rehabilitation, and apply their expertise specifically to stroke rehabilitation or industrial rehabilitation for injured workers. Occupational therapists are also finding new ways of applying their knowledge and skills, such as international practice, universal design, and occupational science. New areas of specialization such as these do not yet have certification programs in place. Certified or not, however, having a specialty is a ticket to open any doorway.

Perhaps the only factor holding back demand for occupational therapy services is related to the ability of patients to pay. Most patients rely on their health insurance to cover expenses. In the past, this was problematic as insurance companies were not ready to pay for people to learn how to do daily tasks. However, times are changing. Federal health insurance reform is making it possible for more people to have access to occupational therapy services. Both rehabilitation and habilitation services are listed among the essential health benefits that insurers will be required to cover.

GETTING STARTED

YOU SHOULD START LAYING THE foundation for your career long before college graduation. Employers not only like to see experience, they expect it – even from newly licensed OTs. One of the best ways to get that experience is through internships. There are many internship programs available through hospitals, rehabilitation centers, nursing homes, and community clinics. Ask your guidance counselor for help finding them. Intern programs typically last about 10 weeks and are usually scheduled during the summer months. Most will not offer compensation, but there are also some that do. Regardless, the goal is to land your first job so try to find out which ones are most likely to lead to job offers after you graduate.

Because internships are so valuable, there can be competition getting into one. In this case, you should seriously consider doing volunteer work. This is actually the most common way aspiring OTs get experience. It will be unpaid work, but it still looks great on a résumé. One big advantage of volunteer work is that it can be found anywhere, even in your hometown when you are home during summer breaks. To find volunteer opportunities, look in the same type of places where you would expect to find internships.

Start networking early. Every contact is valuable, but the best include supervisors from intern or volunteer work and college professors. Networking through the American Occupational Therapy Association is also a good idea.

Decide if you want to specialize in an area such as pediatrics, mental health, or rehabilitation. Knowing your niche is half the work of finding a job. If you are planning on practicing in a big city, you will probably be able to choose a specialty that interests you most. If not, you might have to work as a generalist, for a while at least. Having the additional training and certification in a specialty can only further your career.

Before embarking on your job search, polish your résumé, write a good cover letter, and gather your best references. Looking good on paper is important, but do keep in mind that your greatest asset will be your enthusiasm and your genuine desire to help people.

There are several good places to look for job openings. Your school's career center will certainly have listings. So will the state employment office and the classified section of any newspaper. There are also employment agencies, both on the Internet and off, that specialize in healthcare related jobs. There are professional associations just for occupational therapists that post jobs from all over the country. The American Occupational Therapy Association maintains a job database called OT JobLink.

You do not need to wait for job openings to be advertised. Go straight to the source and apply directly to hospitals, clinics, physicians' offices, school districts, and anywhere else that hires occupational therapists.

While looking for your first job, keep up with advances in occupational therapy through professional journals and conferences, so you are ready to provide high quality patient care.

ASSOCIATIONS

■ **American Occupational Therapy Association**
http://www.aota.org

■ **National Board for Certification in Occupational Therapy**
http://www.nbcot.org

■ **The American Occupational Therapy Foundation**
http://www.aotf.org

PERIODICALS

■ **Advance for Occupational Therapy Practitioners**
http://occupational-therapy.advanceweb.com

■ **The Open Journal of Occupational Therapy**
http://scholarworks.wmich.edu/ojot

WEBSITES

■ **Today in OT**
http://www.todayinot.com

■ **OT JobLink**
http://www.otjoblink.org